Laurent Wendlamita SAWADOGO

Medical responsibility and the influence of medical delegates

Laurent Wendlamita SAWADOGO

Medical responsibility and the influence of medical delegates

in hospital prescribing

ScienciaScripts

Imprint
Any brand names and product names mentioned in this book are subject to trademark, brand or patent protection and are trademarks or registered trademarks of their respective holders. The use of brand names, product names, common names, trade names, product descriptions etc. even without a particular marking in this work is in no way to be construed to mean that such names may be regarded as unrestricted in respect of trademark and brand protection legislation and could thus be used by anyone.

Cover image: www.ingimage.com

This book is a translation from the original published under ISBN 978-620-6-72286-1.

Publisher:
Sciencia Scripts
is a trademark of
Dodo Books Indian Ocean Ltd. and OmniScriptum S.R.L publishing group

120 High Road, East Finchley, London, N2 9ED, United Kingdom
Str. Armeneasca 28/1, office 1, Chisinau MD-2012, Republic of Moldova, Europe
Printed at: see last page
ISBN: 978-620-8-34131-2

Contents

DEDICACES

> **To the Almighty Creator**

Merciful, omnipotent, omnipresent God, I thank you for the graces you have bestowed upon me.

> **To my ancestors**

Thank you for your eternal daily vigil

> **To my late mother ZIDA Antoinette**; who left us very early, we remember you as a woman full of love, fighting spirit, sacrifice and devotion to her children. No words can adequately express your merit. We are grateful for all the suffering you have endured. We hope that through this work you will find all our gratitude for the values that you have instilled in us.

> **To my late father SAWADOGO Yamba Albert;** you were a man of charisma, you lived a useful life. I will be eternally grateful to you for the values you passed on to me. Values to which I was attached throughout my school career. May your soul rest in peace !!!!

> **To my dear uncle Mr SAWADOGO Y Jacques**

The rigorous education we received was simply your desire to see us succeed. May the Almighty grant you health and longevity. AMEN !!!

> **To my brothers and sisters SAWADOGO Pascaline, SAWADOGO Rosalie SAWADOGO Nicolas, SAWADOGO Daniel.**

As a token of the affection that has always united us under my father's roof. I would like you to find in this work the fruit of the sacrifices you have made on my behalf. Let us keep the spirit of family cohesion and the sense of tolerance that our parents instilled in us. This work is also yours. May the Almighty preserve and strengthen our fraternal affection.

> **To my dear aunt Madame ZABA Claudine**

May God grant you health and longevity.

> **To my dear aunt Madame ZIDA Pauline**

I've always seen in you the face of my mother. Thank you for your advice and encouragement.

> **To all other members of the family**

This work is yours. Thank you for your messages and your encouragement.
The good is never lost!!!

> **To my beloved Miss OUEDRAOGO Caroline Wend Neso**

Ever since my second year of medicine, despite the bad weather, you've always found the space and time for me. Thank you for your patience and understanding. May God always keep us together.

> **To my comrades in the struggle at the Faculty of Medicine**

The University has bound us together and we have managed to turn this bond into a fraternity. Thank you !!!! May I mention SAWADOGO Kader, SAVADOGO Kalizeta, SAVADOGO Claude, NARE Guy, SAWADOGO Achille, DIOMA Michel- Ange, SAWADOGO Justine, TRAORE Mohazou, TRAORE Desire, BELEM Aziz, SANOU Dinjin, SANOU Loe. Special mention to members of the KINKELEBA family !!!!

ACKNOWLEDGEMENTS

Our thanks go to :

> **To our thesis supervisor, Doctor W. Norbert RAMDE (MCA), Head of the Forensic Medicine Department at the CHU-BOGODOGO.**

It is a great pleasure and an honour for us that you have agreed to guide us, step by step, in the realisation of this work, despite your multiple occupations. Your simplicity, your modesty, your humility, your availability, your rigour in your work and the breadth of your knowledge make you our reference point. Dear Master, allow us to express to you our deepest gratitude. May God bless you and your family, grant you a successful professional career and shower you with abundant graces! Amen.

> **To Dr. DOUDOULGOU Berare, forensic physician at the CHU BOGODOGO**

Your contribution has been invaluable in the production of this work. Thank you for your availability and we wish you a very good professional and academic career.

> **To Dr. COMPAORE Patrick, forensic physician at the CHU BOGODOGO**

Your contribution to our work has been invaluable. Thank you for your availability and we wish you a very good professional and academic career.

> **To Doctor NAGBILA, internist at the CHU Tengandogo** > **To Doctor SAVADOGO Kalizeta, general practitioner**

> **To Dr Diane Ismaël General Practitioner**

> **To the administrative staff of the UFR/SDS of the Joseph Ki Zerbo University**

You were the ones who gave me my medical training. Thank you very much!

> **To all my teachers at primary, secondary and university level.**

Thank you for the instruction you have given me. I will be eternally grateful. Be honoured.

> **To all those who have supported me in one way or another, may the Lord repay you a hundredfold.**

TO OUR ESTEEMED MASTERS AND JUDGES

To our Master and President of the Jury

Professor Targissus KONSEM,

You are :

- Full professor of stomatology and maxillofacial surgery at the UFR/SDS of the Joseph KI-ZERBO University.
- Stomatologist and maxillo-facial surgeon at the Centre Hospitalier Universitaire Yalgado Ouedraogo (CHU-YO).
- Head of the Stomatology and Maxillofacial Surgery Department at the Centre Hospitalier Universitaire Yalgado Ouedraogo (CHU-YO').
- Head of the Department of Odontostomatology and Maxillofacial Surgery at the Yalgado Ouedraogo University Hospital (CHU-YO);
- Coordinator of the Odontostomatology section of the UFR/SDS of the Joseph KI ZERBO University.
- Coordinator of the DES in Stomatology and Maxillofacial Surgery. Vice-president of the Burkinabe Society of Stomatology and Maxillofacial Surgery.
- General Secretary of the Societe Africaine francophone de S/CMF President of the Societe Savante des sciences de la sante du Burkina Faso
- Chevalier de l'ordre du merite sante.
- Chairman of the CHU/YO medical committee

Dear Maitre, it is a privilege and an honour for us to see you preside over this jury despite your multiple occupations. We have had the grace to benefit from your teaching throughout our university career.

Please accept, Dear Master, the expression of our profound admiration. May God bless you abundantly and give you long life so that present and future generations, here and elsewhere, can benefit from your immense knowledge. AMEN !

To our master and judge

Doctor Welebnoaga Norbert RAMDE

You are :

- Associate Professor of Forensic Medicine at the UFR/SDS of the Joseph KI-ZERBO University
- Diploma in life and health insurance

- Diploma in legal compensation for personal injury ;
- Head of forensic medicine at Bogodogo University Hospital
- Medical expert at the Ouagadougou Court of Appeal

Dear Master,

Your thoroughness, friendliness and easy-going approach have left a lasting impression on us. You are a role model for us.

We would like to thank you for following this long project step by step. In spite of your multiple occupations, you have agreed to direct this work, and we are very grateful to you for this. We appreciate that you are a man of science, available, simple and modest. Your generosity, dynamism and wide-ranging scientific knowledge make you an example to follow. Please allow us to express to you, through this work, our deepest gratitude and respect. May God grant you and your family peace, health, longevity and prosperity. May he assist you in all your activities.

To our master and judge

Doctor Aime Sosthene OUEDRAOGO

You are :

- Associate Professor in Pathological Anatomy and Cytology at the UFR/SDS of the Joseph KI-ZERBO University
- Winner of the prestigious "Andre Gouaze Prize" at the 20th Concours d'Agregation en Medecine, specialising in Anatomy and Pathological Cytology, November 2020, in Brazzaville
- Head of the Pathological Anatomy and Cytology Department at Bogodogo University Hospital
- Doctor-Colonel of the National Armed Forces
- Expert in legal compensation for personal injury

Dear Master

Thank you for agreeing to judge our work.

Your thoroughness, friendliness and easy-going approach have left a lasting impression on us. You are a role model for us.

Please allow us to express our gratitude to you for agreeing to judge our work. We have benefited from your theoretical and practical teaching throughout our university career. We still remember you as a master of knowledge, a man of science, simple and modest. Please accept, dear master, our sincere thanks.

"By deliberation, the Unite de Formation et de Recherche en Science de la Sante (Health Science Training and Research Unit) has decided that the opinions expressed in the essays that will be submitted to it will be taken into account. opinions expressed in the essays to be to be presented must be considered their authors and that that it does not intend to give any approval or disapproval.

INTRODUCTION AND PROBLEM STATEMENT

Prescribing a medical prescription is a major and frequent step in the medical procedure. It must be seen as a specific action taken by doctors on an individual. Choosing the right drug for a given clinical condition is a highly complex process, based on medical knowledge and professional experience [9]. This choice is also made within a socio-economic, legislative and cultural context [9].

Doctors have freedom of prescription in treating patients, but their freedom is limited. When it comes to determining the best treatment for patients, doctors should take into account the cost of the drugs they prescribe in addition to the efficacy and safety of the treatment in question [23]. In fact, prescribing fully engages the prescriber's responsibility. This liability may be criminal, civil or even disciplinary.

The prescriber is responsible for the rational use of medicines; the act of prescribing is part of a relationship of trust between the doctor and the patient. The act of prescribing is part of a relationship of trust between the doctor and the patient. It also involves the provision of correct and comprehensible information in order to obtain free and informed consent. This presupposes that patients receive pharmaceutical products in line with their clinical condition, at doses adapted to their personal needs, for an appropriate duration of treatment, and at the lowest cost to them and their communities [23].

Health professionals play a vital role in ensuring that medicines are used appropriately [3]. Moreover, in recent years, concerns have focused attention on the relationship between prescribers and pharmaceutical companies, in particular the influence of pharmaceutical companies on drug prescribing using promotional tools likely to influence therapeutic choices [3].

The increased dispensing of prescriptions in hospitals, and the incorrect, inadequate, nonsensical or multiple prescribing of antibacterial drugs and injectable products bear witness to the extent of non-rational drug prescribing, especially in primary health care centres [27].

In the pharmaceutical industry, the medical visit accounts for the majority of promotional expenditure (744.15 billion CFA francs), far ahead of digital (10164 billion CFA francs), which nevertheless stands out for its constant dynamism [13]. This budget, dedicated to drug promotion, is divided between

the medical visit, advertising, financing, as well as gifts given directly to prescribers in different ways: official or unofficial [34].
In France, a French study by Regard Citoyen found that the pharmaceutical industry had spent around 159.820 billion CFA francs on gifts to prescribers between January 2012 and June 2014 [27].
Anglo-Saxon studies have shown that prescribers' relationships with the pharmaceutical industry significantly increase non-rational prescribing [34].
In Burkina Faso, the scale of the problem remains unknown. The non-rational prescription of drugs can have consequences for patients in terms of cost and safety of treatment. Microbial resistance to antibiotics may be linked to over-prescription.
The prescriber is responsible for his prescribing and its civil, criminal and disciplinary implications. To our knowledge, no study has been carried out on responsibility in medical prescribing in the face of the influence of medical representatives, hence the interest of our study.

I GENERAL INFORMATION

1. MEDICAL VISIT

1.1 Definition and concept

The medical delegate (DM), also known as medical visitor or medical representative, is defined by article 2 Chapter I of the French Ministry of Health's conditions for the exercise of the profession of medical visitor as: "any natural person employed by a pharmaceutical establishment or a medical promotion agency to present medical and scientific information on a drug or other pharmaceutical product, with a view to its promotion" [25].

The purpose of the medical sales visit is to promote medicines by providing high-quality information and to ensure their correct use by healthcare professionals [1].

A free sample is generally a quantity or packaging of product below the recognised selling price that is offered free of charge to a user [17].

A leaflet is a written document distributed free of charge to encourage readers to take an interest in and buy the product being promoted [17].

A promotional item is an object that generally includes the brand's name and logo and/or is offered to customers (pens, blouses, T-shirts, etc.) [17].

1.2 Roles and training

- **Role of the medical representative**

According to article 13 chapter III of the conditions for practising the profession of medical sales representative issued by the Ministry of Health, the medical sales representative is obliged to provide complete, impartial information that complies with the most recent medical and scientific research data, can be verified and complies with the contents of the marketing authorisation (MA) files for the products being promoted >>[25]. The DM's role is to promote medicinal products, cosmetic products, dietetic products and medical equipment to all healthcare professionals, including pharmacists, parapharmacy managers, dentists, doctors and medical teams working in hospitals, clinics, general or specialist practices and veterinary surgeons. This information must not be based on comparative advantages with similar products or products sharing the same therapeutic indications. They must keep information relating to the samples they hold for traceability purposes, in accordance with the regulations in force. However, it is the doctor's responsibility to ensure the correct use of the medicinal product, to know the place of the medicinal product in the targeted pathology and the recommended therapeutic strategy. This profession may only be practised in

Burkina Faso by persons holding a professional licence issued by the Ministry of Health.

- **Health visitor training**

Basic medical training is not a prerequisite for medical sales representatives. Medical representatives are recruited on the basis of their ability to build relationships with prescribers. Nevertheless, it is worth noting that some medical sales representatives come from paramedical or nursing backgrounds. There are nevertheless medical sales representatives with a medical or pharmacist background, but more often than not it is only with the aim of becoming an executive in the pharmaceutical company [8].

1.3 Communication techniques for medical sales representatives

To communicate more effectively, the medical representative has a wide range of communications equipment to use, including :
free samples: these are free medicines that are usually given to prescribers. Leaflets: these are advertising posters with the logo or name of the promoted drug displayed in consultation offices. Promotional items (prescription pads, pens, gowns, T-shirts, etc.).

- **Main communication**

Drug advertising is governed by the Burkina Faso Public Health Code. Article 2 Chapter I on the conditions for advertising medicines and other pharmaceutical products stipulates that: "Medicine advertising is the information action carried out by a manufacturer, distributor, medical promotion agency or health service provider to encourage the prescription, purchase, consumption and/or request of medicines or other pharmaceutical products >>[26].

Article 4 Chapter I on the conditions for advertising medicines and other pharmaceutical products stipulates that: "Advertising must comply with the relevant regulations in force. In particular, it must be verifiable and not contain allegations or false indications or presentations or be likely to mislead >[26]. Furthermore, advertising for medicinal products for human use means any form of information, including canvassing, canvassing or inducement, which is intended to promote the prescription, supply, sale or consumption of these medicinal products, with the exception of information provided in the course of their duties by pharmacists managing a pharmacy for internal use [7].

- **Medical visit**

The medical sales visit is the pharmaceutical industry's primary means of promoting its products to doctors. It can only be carried out by medical sales representatives who hold a professional licence issued by the Minister of Health. France's Inspectorate General for Social Action (IGAS) states that the principle of the medical sales visit is to meet 5 to 6 doctors a day and present to them the specialities marketed by the firm that employs them [12].

Respecting professional secrecy is a duty of the medical sales representative. The medical representative must also respect the operation of the medical practice, in particular the rhythm and times of visits requested by the doctor, and refrain from denigrating the products of competing companies.

- **Continuing medical education**

Continuing medical education for healthcare workers refers to all the experiences that follow initial training and help healthcare staff to maintain the skills needed to provide healthcare or to acquire new ones. Continuing training therefore encompasses all forms of learning, not just refresher courses, and covers the period from the end of initial training to retirement. It covers not only knowledge but also a wide range of skills that are directly relevant to the provision of healthcare.

Continuing medical education has grown rapidly and now accounts for almost 65% of total revenue from continuing medical education programmes in the USA [33]. Providing financial incentives to CME organisers to create programmes favourable to a company's products is at the root of conflicts of interest. These conflicts arise in medical education and communication companies, many of which are for-profit and are almost exclusively funded by drug and device manufacturers [29]. Some university-based speciality societies and CME providers have provided support for potentially promotional activities.

- **Congress**

Congresses bring together a number of doctors around a theme, with experts in the same speciality taking part. They may or may not be part of a CME programme. Congresses may be organised and financed entirely by the pharmaceutical industry, or they may be organised by learned societies with industrial support. A laboratory may set the programme for a congress if it is the main organiser. The laboratory chooses and pays the participants. The main objective is to provide scientific information for the purposes of continuing medical education, but the promotional role cannot be ignored.

- **Round tables**

Round tables are public discussions led by a moderator, bringing together experts and various people with useful knowledge who can provide information on relevant issues. They are broadly similar to congresses. They may be funded by the pharmaceutical industry as a whole, with a promotional item displayed, and usually end with a snack provided by the pharmaceutical industry.

1.4 . Obligations of the health visitor

The medical sales representative undertakes to exercise his profession with rigour and a sense of responsibility by complying with the rules relating to drug advertising.

and other pharmaceutical products. In this respect, Article 10 Chapter II of the conditions governing advertising of medicines and other pharmaceutical products stipulates that: "the medical representative is prohibited from making the supply of medical samples or any other advantage or benefit conditional on the prescription, dispensing or use of medicinal products by health professionals >>[26].

2. MEDICAL PRESCRIPTION WITH ASSOCIATED FACTORS

2.1 Prescribing rules and associated factors

Medical prescribing, the basis of which is the prescription, is a major medical act based on scientific knowledge and far removed from any kind of personal interest. The prescriber, in his or her efforts to treat, prevent or avoid complications of an illness in his or her patient, has a duty to find the medicines that he or she considers most appropriate in the circumstances and in the patient's best interests. There are several rules to follow when writing a medical prescription.

- **Regulatory information**

The regulatory information that must appear on a prescription is: the date of prescription, the surname, first name and qualification of the prescriber (general practitioner or specialist, dental surgeon, etc.) with the prescriber's signature. The patient's surname, first name, sex and age must also appear on the prescription.

- **Pharmacological information**

The nature of the medicine prescribed, i.e. the brand name or INN; the pharmaceutical form; the dosage; the route of administration; the duration of treatment; and the words 'to be repeated' all need to appear on a medical prescription.

- **Associated factors**

In addition to the knowledge that doctors possess, there are other factors that influence their prescribing decisions. These include university medical training, where the first contact between future prescribers (students) and the pharmaceutical industry takes place. This contact, which is often accompanied by gadgets and meals, is offered to students with the aim of influencing their future therapeutic choices, as indicated by an American study which showed that the offers modified students' prescriptions in favour of these laboratories [30].

Experience is another factor in the choice of medical prescription. According to a New Zealand study, prescribers who had been prescribing for longer had less expensive prescriptions [31].

Doctors who need to keep their knowledge up to date often find new information during continuing medical education courses or medical check-ups. The use of medical representatives would be an easier way of providing therapeutic information.

2.2 Influence of the pharmaceutical industry

Medicines contribute to the day-to-day management of patients. Medicines enable patients to enjoy or maintain good health, but they must be used responsibly. If a patient must have recourse to treatment, they must have access to the best medicines, at an appropriate dosage and for a reasonable length of time [23].

Pharmaceutical industry experts put their activities at the service of patient care: the drug promoted must be the best treatment available [26]. This process is encouraged by marketing techniques. However, in a poly-competitive field where numerous treatments are on the market, pharmaceutical companies are under pressure. All this leads to excessive communication and promotion. Pharmaceutical companies invest exponentially in financial resources. When the budget is drawn up by the laboratory, it is divided between the following means of communication: advertising, the medical press, prescribers' expenses (PEC) at congresses, samples, public relations and medical visits. The medical delegate provides doctors with materials in the form of drug samples, scientific books, medical equipment, invitations to social or educational events, etc.

Eurostaf-Direct Medica carried out a survey in 2008 which found that "88 billion dollars were spent on pharmaceutical promotion, broken down as follows [11] :

- Medical check-up
- Drug samples
- Meetings
- Direct to consumer

- Advertising

On the other hand, any prescriber can be influenced by the promotional techniques used by the pharmaceutical industry, and usually the prescriber is unaware of this influence. Prescribers are people like any other, working in other areas of life. Evidence exists that exposure to pharmaceutical company promotion has a real influence on medical practice and prescribing patterns [21]. In other words, gifts do influence behaviour, despite the widespread belief among prescribers that they are personally invulnerable to such attention [35].

Many prescribers, who accept materials in kind or in cash as gifts from pharmaceutical companies, are convinced that pharmaceutical promotion influences patient management, even though several studies have proved the opposite [3].

Men can be grateful for gestures of attention and generosity, especially when they feel it is deserved, given their commitment to the profession, which is often linked to what they feel is insufficient recognition [3]. It goes without saying that the gifts received by prescribers give rise to a feeling of reciprocity, of giving something in return. The pharmaceutical industry provides many types of gifts to healthcare professionals, including medical students [2]: pens, meals, medical equipment, continuing medical education (CME), research funding, consultants' or speakers' fees^ and even trips to the most distant countries and islands, or even cheques and vouchers.

However, in the face of this practice, many pharmaceutical companies have been found guilty of corruption and have had to pay fines:

> Between 2006 and 2014, pharmaceutical companies were implicated in cases of corruption in Greece. The Novartis pharmaceutical industry was implicated [18]. Novartis also experienced a similar case in 2016 in Turkey, South Korea and the USA [15].

> GSK has also been implicated in similar cases in China. It is alleged to have bribed doctors to prescribe its drugs, or in the USA [19]. This laboratory paid $3 billion in damages to the US administration.

> The major Israeli pharmaceutical company Teva paid $520 million for bribing prescribers in Russia, Ukraine and Mexico [20].

2.3 Medical responsibility in prescribing

The choice of appropriate treatment presupposes a correct diagnosis. While any error in diagnosis does not constitute a fault, the choice of treatment can. However, doctors are free to choose the treatment they wish, as stipulated in

article 11 of the code of ethics for doctors in Burkina Faso, which states that: "Doctors are free to prescribe as they wish, but they must take account of their duty to provide moral assistance and limit their prescriptions and actions to what is necessary for the quality, safety and effectiveness of care" [27].
When prescribing medicines, doctors have a duty to find the best treatment for their patients. He must take into account the cost, efficacy and safety of the treatment in question. To find the best treatment, according to the Ontario Council's report, several values must be considered [23] :

> Sustainability: the drugs programme and, more broadly, our healthcare system must provide quality care within reasonable public budget limits. To achieve this, it is essential to take account of the price of drugs.

> Shared responsibility: healthcare providers share responsibility for managing the costs of the healthcare system. This also includes the cost of medicines.

> Impartiality and fairness: as far as the budget allows, all citizens should have access to the medicines they need. Consequently, the members of the Council believe that it is acceptable to limit individual choice in order to be able to offer a greater number of medicines, within the same budget envelope, to those who need them.

> Evidence-based decision-making: the members of the board felt that safety and efficacy are the characteristics to be considered as a priority when it comes to drugs. However, when certain drugs show similar clinical results, cost must become a factor to be considered. This latter value has proved essential in order to qualify the cost factor and focus instead on cost-effectiveness. In this case, it is the drug that provides equivalent results at the lowest cost. This led to the formulation of the following key principle:
When pharmacological treatments are therapeutically equivalent (sufficiently similar clinical results) in terms of efficacy and safety, the most cost-effective drug (lowest cost for equivalent results) should be prescribed first. In the same report, the members tried to put themselves in the place of prescribers by illustrating the figure below:

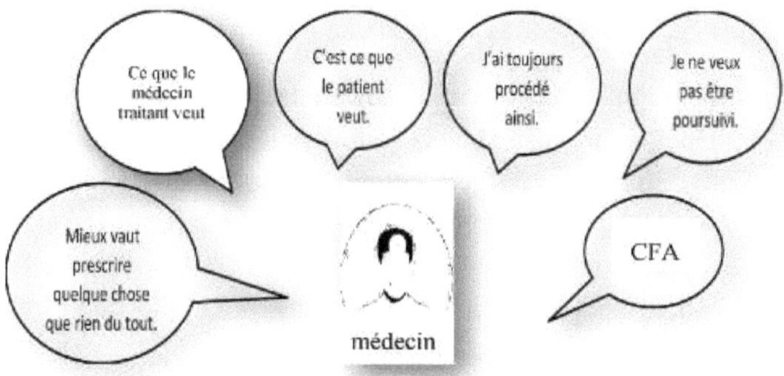

Figure 1: Prescriber's set of imaginative questions [23].

The doctor is a citizen who carries out a risky activity within an organised profession. If he commits a fault in the exercise of his art, he may be punished by the professional courts (disciplinary) or by the ordinary courts (civil or criminal).

> **Civil liability**

Civil liability relates to actions committed in the context of a liberal medical practice, including an activity, clinic, dispensary, health centre, or at the hospital in the context of a private practice [24]. Medical civil liability is a matter for the tribunal de grande instance and the cour d'appel: the penalties are financial [24]. Despite the doctor's therapeutic freedom, as stipulated in article 11 of the code of ethics for doctors: "The doctor is free to prescribe as he wishes, but he must take account of his duty to provide moral assistance and limit his prescriptions and actions to what is necessary for the quality, safety and effectiveness of care"[28]. The fact remains that a doctor cannot, on pain of incurring civil liability, recommend any treatment whatsoever. He will be liable if he chooses a method that a normally prudent and diligent doctor in the same circumstances would not have chosen. His civil liability may be incurred in full if the doctor prescribes medication to his patient without taking into account the side effects, or by prolonging the duration of treatment, or by deliberately exceeding the recommended dose in order to induce the patient to use several boxes for the benefit of the pharmaceutical companies. Liability may also arise where prescribing is inappropriate, i.e. excessive prescribing, for example in the case of double prescribing of the same therapeutic class.

> **Criminal liability**

Criminal liability is the obligation to answer for offences committed and to undergo the punishment provided for by the text that punishes it. Medical malpractice is judged by the police courts for minor offences, the criminal divisions of the high courts for misdemeanours and the assize court for felonies [24]. Doctors are also subject to this obligation, and in the event of misconduct they may be charged before the criminal courts, tried and possibly sentenced to a fine and/or a custodial sentence. In the context of prescribing, such misconduct may include a deliberate breach of a safety or prudence obligation, i.e. prescribing a drug that is not authorised by the MA, or an infringement of drug legislation.

> **Disciplinary liability**

Disciplinary liability is a responsibility imposed on all persons to answer for their actions before the authority on which they depend [17]. Disciplinary medical liability is the responsibility of the Burkina Faso Order of Physicians. Misconduct that may give rise to disciplinary liability may include prescribing medication that is not safe for the patient, i.e. medication that could have a negative impact on the patient. Other examples of misconduct include ineffective or unqualified prescribing. The Ordre des Medecins reserves the right to sanction any doctor in the event of professional misconduct or any misconduct deemed inappropriate. Penalties may range exponentially, from a warning to blame, or from temporary striking off to permanent striking off.

PART II: OUR STUDY

OBJECTIVES

1. OBJECTIVES

1. **1. General objective**

To study the responsibility of doctors in the face of the influence of medical representatives on medical prescribing in hospitals from December 2023 to January 2024 in Ouagadougou.

2. **2. Specific objectives**
3. Describe the socio-professional characteristics of prescribers
4. Determine the daily attendance rate of doctors by medical representatives.
5. Identify the type of information provided by visitors to prescribers.
6. Identify the influence of medical representatives on medical prescribing.
7. To assess doctors' knowledge of prescribing responsibility as influenced by visits from medical representatives.

METHODOLOGY

2. METHODOLOGY

2.1. Scope of the study

The study was carried out in public hospitals in Ouagadougou, Burkina Faso.

2.1.1. Organisation of the health system in Burkina Faso

Public health services in Burkina Faso are organised operationally on a pyramid structure comprising three levels providing primary, secondary and tertiary health care. The first level corresponds to the health district and comprises two levels: Medical Centre with Surgical Antenna (CMA), Health and Social Promotion Centre (CSPS). The second level corresponds to the regional hospital centre (CHR), which serves as a reference and referral centre for the CMA, and the third level to the university hospital centres (CHU) [26].

University hospitals and medical centres with a surgical branch are places where the number of prescriptions is high and where medical representatives are more frequent, hence the interest of our study in these different sites.

Ouagadougou has four university hospitals, including the

- TENGANOGO University Hospital
- CHU YALGADO OUEDRAOGO
- CHU BOGODOGO
- CHU CHARLES DE GAULLE

It also has five medical centres with surgical facilities

- CMA of KOSSODO
- PISSY CMA
- CMA of BOGODOGO
- PAUL VI HOSPITAL
- BASKUY CMA
- SCHIPHRA HOSPITAL

2.2. Type and period of study

This was a quantitative, descriptive, cross-sectional study. Data collection began on 08 January and ended on 31 January 2024.

2.3. Study population

Our study population consisted of doctors working in public health centres in the city of Ouagadougou.

> **Inclusion criteria**

Our study included :

Doctors in Ouagadougou who have given their consent.

> **Non-inclusion criteria**

Not included in this study:

Private sector doctors.

Doctors who have not given their consent.

2.4. Sampling

> **Sample size**

This was a probabilistic and systematic sampling of the simple random type. All the lists of doctors in public facilities in the city of Ouagadougou were compiled into a single list numbered from 1 to N. Let n be the size of our sample.

n= 1.96" 2 x (P) (1-P) / d 2

1.96 = Z for p=0.05 or 95% CI

P= proportion found in Mali = 83.3%.

d = desired precision (0.05 for ± 5%)

n= 1.96^2 x (0.83 (1-O.83) / 0.05^2

n= 213cas

Assuming 10% non-respondents, n=235

According to the HRDs of the various public bodies, the number of doctors in the city of Ouagadougou was 1,294.

Given the number N, the size of the population and n the size of the

In the sample, the pitch was 6

We chose the number at random and drew the sample systematically with one step.

2.5. Variables

Variables	Types	Details
Socio-professional characteristics of the		**prescriber**
Age	Quantitative discrete	In years
Gender	Nominal quantity	1. Male 2. Female
Health establishment	Nominal quantity	1. CHU 2. CMA

Doctor's qualifications	Nominal quantity	1. Specialist 2. Specialisation 3. Generalist
Old	Quantitative discrete	In years
Frequent visits by medical representatives to health centres		
Medical visit	Binary qualitative	1. Yes 2. No
Number of daily visits	Quantitative discrete	Natural whole
Time passes	Quantitative discrete	In minutes
Weekly laboratory visits	Quantitative discrete	Natural whole
Quality of exchanges between medical representatives and doctors		
Basic profession of the D.M	Nominal quantity	1. Doctor 2. Pharmacist 3. Nurse 4. Don't know 5. Other
Presents regus	Binary qualitative	1. Yes 2. No
Present type	Nominal quantity	1. Medical equipment 2. Silver 3. Drug samples 4. Fuel 5. Catering 6. Congress 7. Other
Verification of information	Binary qualitative	1. Yes 2. No
Origin of information verification	Nominal quantity	1. Colleagues 2. Reading articles 3. Other
Type of information	Nominal quantity	1. Dosage 2. Dosage 3. Side effects

		4. Duration of treatment 5. Shapes 6. Efficiency 7. Prices
Form of the medicine	Nominal quantity	1. Injectables 2. Tablets 3. Topicals 4. Other
Drug class	Nominal quantity	1. Antibiotics 2. Anti-inflammatory 3. Analgesics 4. Other
Prescription-related factors		
Number of prescriptions	Quantitative discrete	As a natural number
Type of prescription	Nominal quantity	1. DCI 2. Speciality
Influence of D.M	Binary qualitative	1. Yes 2. No
Source of information on new drugs	Binary qualitative	1. Yes 2. No
Limitation period following a promise	Binary qualitative	1. Yes 2. No
Refusal of offers	Binary qualitative	1. Yes 2. No
Type of liability	Nominal quantity	1. Civil 2. Penale 3. Administrative 4. Disciplinary
Faults attributable to civil liability	Nominal quantity	1. Non-compliant prescription 2. Incorrect dosage/route of administration 3. Contraindications 4. Failure to monitor
Fault attributable to criminal liability	Nominal quantity	1. Deliberate failure to observe a duty of safety or care 2. Infringement of medicines

		legislation 3. Overdosing
Fault attributable to disciplinary liability	Nominal quantity	1. Prescription not effective 2. Unqualified prescription 3. Non-secure prescription
Penalties provided for by the French Medical Association	Nominal quantity	1. The warning 2. The blame 3. Temporary deregistration 4. Permanent deregistration

2.6. Data collection and processing

> Collection tools/instruments

Data collection forms were designed and deployed using KoboCollect software. The data was collected physically by proposing and filling in a form offered to the doctors, while preserving confidentiality and anonymity. We then manually inserted the data collected from the doctors on the koboCollect platform.

> Data source

Specialist doctors
Doctors in specialisations
General practitioners

> Data processing

The data collected physically was exported in Excel and world format and analysed using EPI Info statistical data processing software version 7.2.2.6.
The dependent and independent variables have been summarised in the form of averages or percentages, or in graphical form. Categorical variables are presented as frequencies and percentages.

2.7. Ethical and deontological considerations

Our study was submitted for authorisation to the general directors of the university hospital centres in Ouagadougou and also to the regional director of health for the centre for collection in the medical centres with surgical units in Ouagadougou. Confidentiality and anonymity were maintained throughout the data collection process until the results were available.

RESULTS

3. RESULTS

A total of 213 doctors working in public hospitals in Ouagadougou were interviewed for the study.

3.1. Socio-professional characteristics of the prescriber

Breakdown of prescribers by age

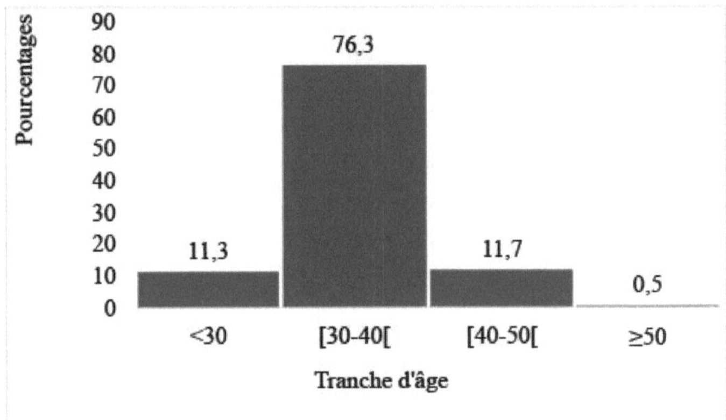

Figure 2: proportion of prescribers by age group

The 30-40 age group accounted for 76.3%.

- **Gender breakdown of prescribers**

Males accounted for 58.7% of the total, giving a sex ratio of 1.42.

Breakdown of prescribers by type of healthcare establishment

We recorded 65.3% of doctors in university hospitals and 34.7% in medical centres with surgical units.

- **Breakdown of prescribers by professional qualification**

Figure 3 shows the breakdown by prescriber qualification.

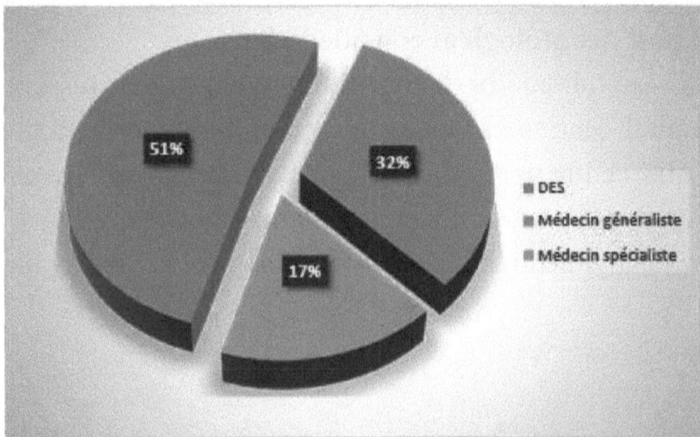

Figure 3: Proportion of prescribers by qualification

Specialist doctors accounted for 51% of our prescribers.

- Breakdown of prescribers by speciality

General practitioners accounted for 32% or 68.

A breakdown of prescribers by speciality is shown in table I.

Table I: Proportion of prescribers by speciality

Speciality	Workforce n=145	Percentages (%)
Medicine	**62**	**42,8**
Surgery	46	31,7
Gynecology	15	10,3
Paediatrics	22	15,2
Total	**145**	**100**

Prescribers of medical specialities accounted for 42.8%.

- Breakdown of prescribers by seniority

. A breakdown of prescribers according to their length of time in medicine is shown in figure 4.

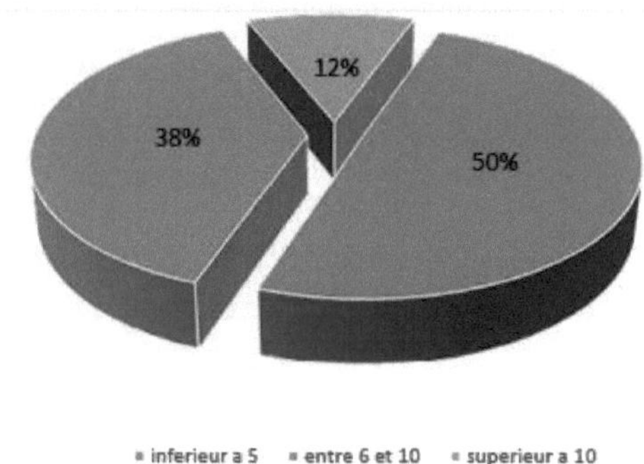

Figure 4: proportion of prescribers by age

Prescribers with less than five years' experience accounted for 50%.

3.2. Frequent visits by medical representatives to health centres

- **Medical visit**

95.8% of doctors say they have already received a visit from at least one medical representative.

- **Breakdown by number of daily visits**

4.23% or 9 doctors refused the medical visit.

95.77% or 204 doctors agreed to receive the medical delegates

Table II shows the breakdown by number of daily visits.

Table I: Proportion of prescribers according to the number of regular daily visits

Number of visits	Number n=204	Percentages (%)
[1-2]	**176**	**86,3**
[3-4]	21	10,3
> 5	7	3,4
Total	**204**	**100**

86.3% of prescribers admit to one or two visits a day.

- Breakdown by time spent with delegates

90.2% of prescribers spent less than 10 minutes during a visit with delegates. The time spent with a delegate varied between one minute and 30 minutes.

3.3. Quality of exchanges between medical representatives and doctors

- **Breakdown by type of gift received from the medical representative**

Table III shows the distribution of prescribers according to the nature of the drugs prescribed.

Table III: Breakdown of prescribers by nature of prescriptions received

Presents regus	Numbers (n=194)	Percentages (%)
Drug samples	**178**	**91,8**
Medical equipment	169	87,1
Catering	77	39,7
Conference funding	76	39,2
Fuel	22	11,3
Silver	43	22,2
Credits unite	14	7,2
Internet connection	3	1,5
Gadget	2	1,0
Television subscription	1	0,5

91.8% of prescribers received drug samples.

- **Breakdown of prescribers according to the source of information given by the medical representatives.**

13.26% (27 doctors) did not check the information given by the medical representative.

86.76% or 177 doctors checked the information given by the medical delegate.

A breakdown of prescribers according to the source of verification of the information given by the medical delegate is shown in table V.

Table IV: source of verification of 1 information

Sources of verification	**Workforce (n=177)**	**Percentages (%)**
Internet	**78**	**44,1**
Colleague	60	33,9
Read article	54	30,5
Information leaflet	26	14,7
Vidal	12	6,8

In 44.1% of cases, the internet was used to verify the information provided by the medical representative.

- **Breakdown according to the class of drug most frequently prescribed.**

A breakdown by drug class is shown in Figure 5.

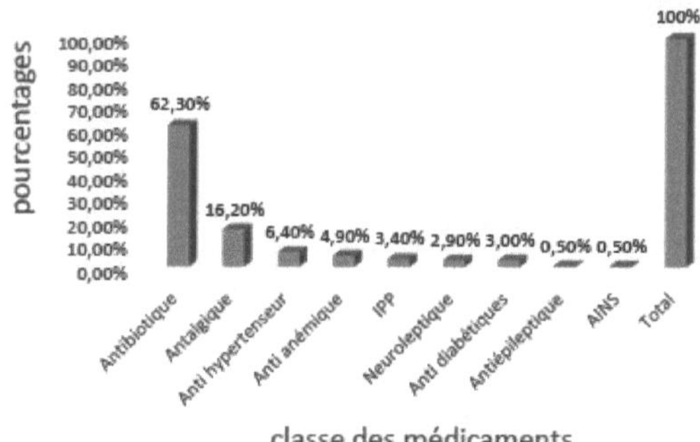

Figure 5: Proportion according to the class of drug most frequently prescribed Antibiotics accounted for 62.3%.

3.4. Prescription-related factors

- Proportion by type of molecule prescribed

A breakdown of prescribers by type of specialty is shown in Figure 6.

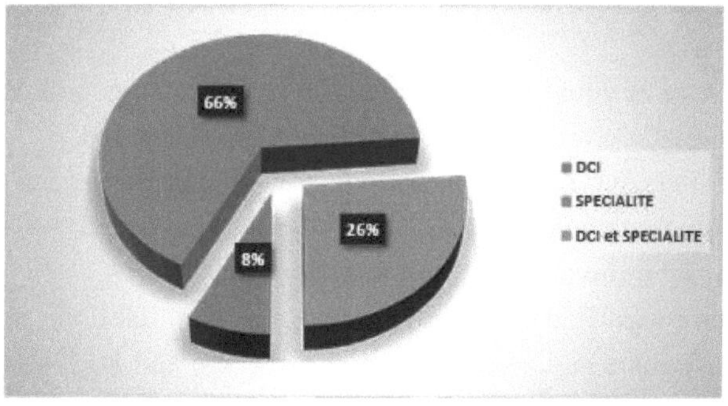

Figure 6: Proportion by type of prescription

Prescribers used speciality drugs in 66% of cases.

- Recognition of the influence of medical representatives on medical prescriptions

81.7% of prescribers acknowledged the influence of medical representatives on their prescribing.

- Proportion of reasons for refusal cited by doctors

83.8 of doctors said they accepted offers from medical representatives. Those who refused represented 16.2%.

The reasons given for refusal are illustrated in Figure 7.

reason for refusal

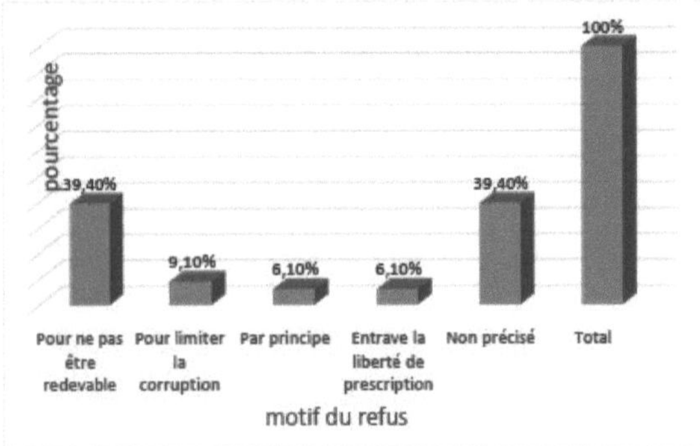

Figure 7: Breakdown by reason for refusal

83.9 % of prescribers said that the reason for their refusal was that they were not liable for payment.

- **Prescribers' knowledge of the type of liability incurred by the prescription**

To assess prescribers' knowledge of the type of liability incurred by prescribing, we gave a score of 5 for each correct answer and 0 for each incorrect answer.

Any mark above or equal to the average (10) constituted good knowledge and any mark below the average (10) constituted bad knowledge.

Of the prescribers surveyed, 15% had a below-average score and 85% had an average or above-average score.

- **Prescribers' knowledge of civil liability**

The same score was used to assess knowledge of civil liability.

19.9% of prescribers had a score below the average and 80.1% of prescribers had a score equal to or above the average.

- Knowledge of criminal liability

23.4 % of prescribers had a score below average and 76.6% had a score equal to or above average.

- Knowledge of disciplinary liability

34.7 % of prescribers had a score below average and 65.3% had a score equal to or above average.

- Knowledge of the sanctions provided for by the French Medical Association (ordre des medecins)

12.6% of doctors scored below average and 87.4% of doctors scored at or above average.

- Total score for assumption of medical responsibility for prescribing

Medical responsibility for prescribing in general was assessed by adding up all the scores and averaging 50 points.

21.12% of doctors had a score below the average and 78.88% of doctors had a score above or equal to the average.

COMMENT/DISCUSSION

4. COMMENT/DISCUSSION

This cross-sectional study involved 138 doctors specialising in 68 general practitioners and 36 specialists, including 139 from university hospitals and 74 from medical centres with surgical units, with the aim of describing the influence of medical representatives and assessing the responsibility of prescribers in the face of this influence. In a health centre, doctors are encouraged to provide quality care and to use pharmaceutical products efficiently and rationally. The prescribing physician, faced with a multitude of information about the drug, must always be faithful to medical ethics while putting the patient's interests first. The doctor can be influenced by all sorts of means on the part of a medical representative. The prescriber assumes professional responsibility.

This study of responsibility in prescribing was subject to certain classic limitations and constraints.

4.1. Limits and constraints of our study

By its very nature, this study was subject to classic biases and limitations:

> Incorrect transmission of certain information

> The non-involvement of medical representatives and pharmacies in the study

> Male collection forms completed by prescribers

4.2. Socio-professional characteristics

The majority of prescribers (76.3%) were aged between 30 and 40. This result is much better than that of A. TRAORE (Mali 2023) who found 57.1% for an age range between 30 and 40 years [33]. This proportion could be explained by the fact that our study focused more on doctors specialising in this field. Doctors specialising in this field represent a young class, as does the predominantly young population of Burkina Faso.

Of the doctors surveyed, 65.3% came from university hospitals and 34.7% from medical centres with surgical units. This could be explained by the fact that the university hospitals are the reference centres for the city of Ouagadougou, where a high number of doctors can be found. The university role of these centres makes them the training ground for DESs, who represented a large proportion of our sample.

Our prescribers with less than 5 years' professional experience were the most represented (50%). This can be explained by the fact that doctors in specialisation represented more than 51.2% and had an average age of between 30 and 40. Doctors in specialisation most often took up specialisation 2 to 3 years after completing their studies.

4.3. Frequent visits to hospitals

In 95.8% of cases, our prescribers stated that they had received at least one medical visit during their career. This result is comparable to that found by A. TRAORE (Mali 2023) who found 92.9% [33]. This proportion could be explained by the fact that the pharmaceutical industry uses the medical visit as the main means of promoting medicines [33].

Doctors 86.3% said they received between 1 and 2 visits a day and spent less than 10 minutes with a medical representative. This result is far superior to that of A. TRAORE who found that 52.3% of prescribers received between 1 and 2 visits per day and spent more than 10 minutes during a visit [33]. A study carried out in Tunisia by Salaheddine R found that 10% of GPs reported receiving visits from pharmaceutical representatives on a daily basis [5]. This result could be explained by the fact that our study took place in hospitals. Hospitals are centres where the daily prescriptions are enormous and the frequency of visits by medical representatives is high. A. TRAORE's study took place in a community health centre.

4.4. Quality of discussions between medical representative and doctor

In our study, drug samples represented 91.8% of gifts received. This result is higher than that found by Campbell and Parker (USA 2005), which was 80% of drug samples received [6]. This could be explained by the fact that pharmaceutical promotion in our context is fairly advanced and uncontrolled. Burkina Faso is also a poor country where medicines are expensive. These drug samples are also used by doctors to give to needy patients or to sell.

Medical equipment came second as a gift offered to prescribers with 87.1%. These results could be explained by the fact that pharmaceutical marketing uses the lack of medical equipment in hospitals to better influence prescribers. This material, almost always containing special logos or acronyms, is a daily reminder to doctors of the incentive to prescribe. In our study, attendance at congresses financed by pharmaceutical companies accounted for 39.7%. This result for congress attendance is similar to that found by Campbell and Parker 40% [6] but lower than that found by F. SANGHO (Mali 2018) which was 61.1% [32]. This proportion can be explained by the fact that attendance at congresses is more common among specialists, and in our study specialists were outnumbered by general practitioners and specialists.

In our study, 86.77% of our prescribers verified the information given by the medical representative, compared with 13.23% who did not. In our study, the Internet was the main source of information for our doctors, with a percentage of 44.1%, followed by checking information with colleagues (33.9%), reading articles (30.5%), leaflets (14.7%), Vidal (6.8%), whereas F. Sangho found that 62.9% [32] stated that their source of information was personal studies carried out on the drug. This could be explained by the fact that our prescribers were in the city of Ouagadougou with an available and accessible internet connection.
Antibiotics were the class of drug most frequently presented, with a rate of 62.3%. This result is higher than that found by F. SANGHO who found 55.6% [32]. This can be explained by the high frequency of bacterial infections and perhaps the irrational use of antibiotics in our context, so the emphasis seems to be on promoting antibiotics.

4.5. Limitation period and liability

A predominance of speciality prescriptions representing 66% was found. This result is lower than that found by F. SANGHO, which was 84.1% [32]. This proportion could be explained by the fact that our study included the gynaecology and paediatrics departments, where there is free care for pregnant women and children under 5 years of age, with the prescription of recommended generic drugs.
In our study, 81.7% of doctors acknowledged the influence of delegates on their prescribing. This result is similar to that of F. SANGHO, who found a rate of 83.3% [32]. In contrast, a German study found that only 34% of prescribers thought they were influenced by delegates [30]. This could be explained by the low income of our prescribers compared with German prescribers.
More than half of our prescribers (53.9%) find out about new medicines during medical visits. This high priority given to
to the delegate has been documented by a study which states that the medical visit is an indispensable source of information [20].
For each type of responsibility, a score of 0 to 20 was used for re-evaluation. Any score below 10 constituted poor knowledge, while any score of 10 or more constituted good knowledge. This score showed that 15% of prescribers had poor knowledge of the type of medical liability incurred by the prescription, while 85% had good knowledge of these types of liability. The majority of our prescribers had good knowledge. This may be due to the presence of continuing medical education.

In our study, the same score was used to determine our prescribers' knowledge of civil liability. Our results showed that 19.9% of prescribers had poor knowledge compared with 80.1% who had good knowledge of civil liability. A prescriber's criminal liability may result in varying penalties depending on the nature of the offence. The penalty of deprivation of liberty, which may vary in length, may be accompanied by fines ranging from imprisonment to a fine. In our study of criminal liability, 23.4% of prescribers had poor knowledge, compared with 76.6% who had good knowledge of criminal liability. Disciplinary liability was also studied and with the same score 34.7% had poor knowledge while 65.3% had good knowledge of disciplinary liability. In the event of such liability being incurred, the Ordre des medecins reserves the right to initiate disciplinary proceedings. Doctors' knowledge of the penalties incurred showed that 34.7% had poor knowledge compared with 65.3% who had good knowledge of the penalties incurred. Knowledge of all the medical responsibilities involved in prescribing under the influence studied showed that

78.88% had good knowledge and 21.1% had poor knowledge. This state of affairs can be explained by the fact that, firstly, during the university training of doctors, there are courses on the responsibility of the doctor in his or her profession, and secondly by the presence of continuing medical education, and also by the fact that our study mainly concerned doctors in specialisation, who receive continuing courses on forensic medicine during their specialisation.

CONCLUSION

Good prescribing habits and the appropriate use of prescription drugs are an important factor in maintaining the excellence and viability of our healthcare system. Our study has shown us the effective influence of visits by medical representatives on prescribing in hospitals. The vast majority of our doctors acknowledged the influence of pharmaceutical representatives on their prescribing. Free samples, medical equipment and attendance at congresses were the most common gifts offered to prescribers by pharmaceutical company representatives. This study showed that doctors in specialties received medical sales representatives more frequently.

Prescribers need to be aware of this influence and their responsibility for it. The study of responsibility in prescribing has revealed shortcomings in prescribers who act or prescribe without knowing the risks involved and the penalties provided for. The judge or the medical association are the bodies responsible for applying penalties to prescribers. No one is deemed to be ignorant of the law, and doctors cannot rely on ignorance of the responsibility involved in prescribing medication as an argument in their defence before the competent courts. It is the doctor's duty to inform himself and to remain faithful to the texts governing the medical profession.

SUGGESTIONS

At the end of our study, we have a few suggestions:

Health facilities:

> Regulating the access of medical visitors to health facilities

> Establish rules for the visit so as not to inconvenience prescribers and their patients

Prescribers:

> Intensify continuing medical training for staff

> Avoid drawing up contracts with pharmaceutical representatives

> Putting the patient's interests first in terms of effective prescribing

Medical visitors:

> To respect the rules of medical ethics and deontology

> To comply with regulations governing medical promotion

> Complying with regulations in the role of medical representative

> Avoid drawing up contracts with prescribers

REFERENCES

1. **Acceuil B.** Les Entreprises du Medicament - Who are we ? [Internet]. Available at: https://www.leem.org/les-entreprises-du-medicament-qui-about us . [consulted on 4 Jan 2024]

2. **Austad K, Avorn J, Kesselheim S**. Medical Students' Exposure to and Attitudes about the Pharmaceutical Industry: A Systematic Review. PLoS Med. 2011;8(5).P-21

3. **Barbara M, Dee M, Hayes L**. Understanding pharmaceutical promotion: state of the art in teaching postgraduate and postgraduate general medical students. 2017;

4. **Baumann S, Braudo S,** Civil liability - Definition . Legal Dictionary. 2024

5. **Ben A, Harrabi I, Rahmani S, Ghedira A, Gaha K, Ghannem H**. [Attitudes of general practitioners to pharmaceutical sales representatives in Sousse]. East Mediterr Health J. 2003;9(5-6): 1075-83.

6. **Campbell J., Parker M. and Ten Bos R**. Business Ethics.A Critical Approach", New York, Routledge, 2005.

7. **French Public Health Code**. Decree n°2023-1371 of 28 December 2023. Chapter III L. 5213-1 p130 - 3876.

8. **Medical delegate - medical representative - medical visitor** [Internet]. [consulted on 19 Jan 2024]. Available from: https://www.pharmapro.ch/fr/N16677/delegue-medical.html

9. **Marco V**. Ecouter Penser Parler Rev Med Suisse.2008.4.174.2182 p 4.

10. **Foisset E**. SPECIALITE: Medecine Generale [These] : etude de 1 impact de la visite medicale sur la qualité des prescriptions des medecins generalistes bretons. thesis N°2912002. [BREST]: universite de bretagne occidentale; 2012.

11. **Haute autorite de sante**. Charte de la visite medicale. France 2009; p54.

12. **IGAS**. Promotion des medicaments en France. sept 2008;(299):704-5.

13. **IQVIA** Drug promotion: is it time for digital? - [Internet]. [Accessed 6 Jan 2024]. Available from: https://www.iqvia.com/fr-en/locations/france/newsroom/2018/12/promotion-du-medicament

14. **Kobryner A**. Le medecin generaliste et la prescription medicamenteuse. Nancy. 1993;

15. **La Presse**. Investigation into Norvatis. La Presse. 1 Jul 2020; Available at:

https://www.lapresse.ca/affaires/entreprises/2020-07-01/pots-de-vin-novartis-accept-to-pay-over-642-millions-us.php Accessed 01 Feb 2024
16. Available at :https://lumassan-france.fr/burkinafaso/santeburkina.html. Accessed on 20 Jan 2024
17. **Larousse**. Definitions - Dictionnaire de frangais Larousse edition 2022
18. **Le Figaro**. Medicines: Grace claims 214 million euros from Novartis. Le Figaro. 2022. Available at: https://www.lefigaro.fr/flash-eco/medicaments-la-grece-reclame-214-millions-d-euros-a-novartis-20220617 Accessed 19 Jan 2024
19. **Le Monde.fr**. Corruption: GSK admits offences in France China. Available at: https://www.lemonde.fr/economie/article/2013/07/23/corruption-le-laboratoire- gsk-reconnait-des-infractions-en-chine_3451437_3234.html
20. **Le Monde.fr**. Teva, the world's number one in generics, convicted of corruption [Internet]. [cited 21 dec 2023]. Available from: https://www.lemonde.fr/entreprises/article/2018/01/15/teva-le-numero-un-mondial-des-medicaments-generiques-condamne-pour-corruption_5242001_1656994.html [Accessed 19 Jan 2024].
21. **Lexchin J**. What information do physicians receive from pharmaceutical representatives? Can Fam Physician. May 1997;43:941-5.
22. **Lieb K, Scheurich A**. Contact between Doctors and the Pharmaceutical Industry, Their Perceptions, and the Effects on Prescribing Habits. PLoS ONE. 16 Oct 2014;9(10):e110130.
23. **McGurn S**. Ontario citizens' council report health system renewal. 2015; p17-36
24. **Bernard M.** 160 Questions en responsabilite medicale 2° edition (Masson) 2010. p 9 . p 10
25. **Ministere de la sante** decret portant condition de 1'exercice de la profession de visiteur medicale du ministere de la sante. july 17, 2017 p. 7.
26. **Ministere de la sante**. conditions de la publicité sur les medicaments et other pharmaceutical products Burkina Faso.7 fevr, 2017.
27. **Mohamed S**. THESIS: Influence of pharmaceutical companies' marketing practices on the ethics of the medical function in Morocco . MOROCCO Mohamed V University Rabat; 2018
28. **Ordre des medecins du Burkina**. Decree n° 2014-048/pres/ pm/ms portant code de deontologie des medecins du Burkina Faso. fevr p. 2. 55
29. **Steinbrook R**, M.D. Commercial Support and Continuing Medical Education. 2005. 535 p.

30. **Rugmini W**. Do drug samples influence resident prescribing behaviour? 2016 March p. 8. Report No.: 4.
31. **Salisbury C, Bosanquet N, Wilkinson E, Bosanquet A**, Hasler J. The implementation of evidence-based medicine in general practice prescribing. Br J Gen Pract. Dec 1998;48(437):1849-52.
32. **Sangho F, Diop AT, Sangho A, Sangho O, Dianguina S, Arama D, Coulibaly Y, Toure M, Soucko KA, Bah S**. [These] : effet de la visite des delegues medicaux sur la prescription au chu du point g. 2021;
33. **Traore A.** [These] contribution des visiteurs medicaux dans l information pharmaceutique des prescripteurs de la commune rurale de Kalaban-Coro (Kati) USTTB; 2023
34. **Troyen A.** Health Industry Practices That Create Conflicts of Interest. 25 May 2006;5.
35. **Zipkin D, Steinman M**. Interactions Between Pharmaceutical Representatives and Doctors in Training. J Gen Intern Med. August 2005;20(8):777-86.

ICONOGRAPHY

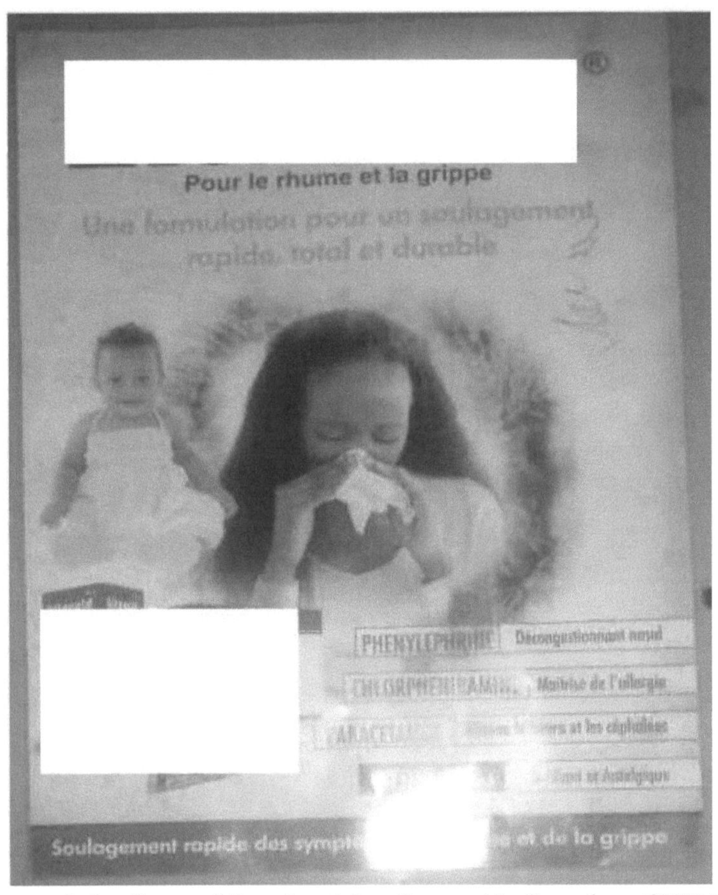

Image 1: Leaflet used for advertising. Source (L. Sawadogo CHU-B)

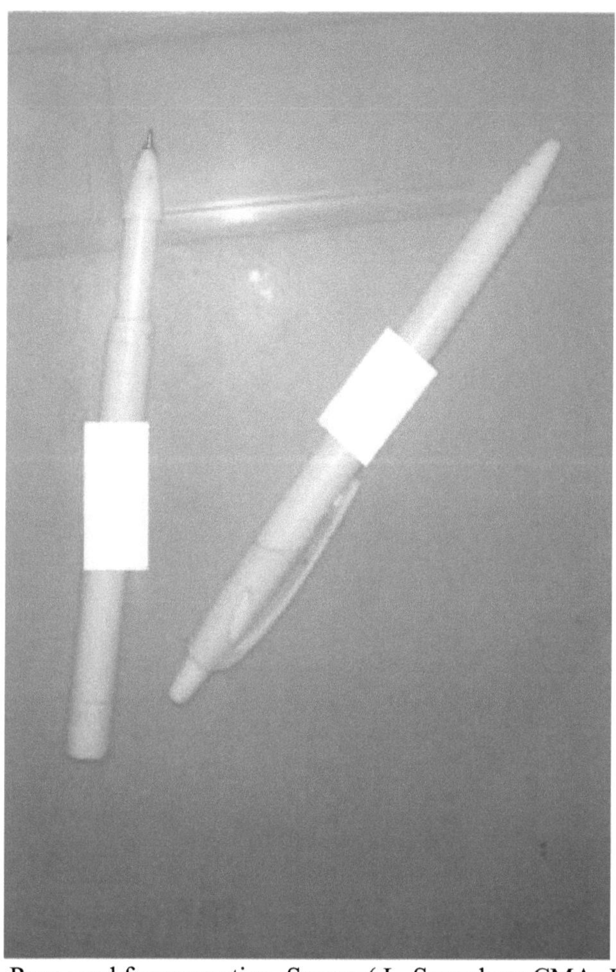

Image 2: Pens used for promotion. Source (L. Sawadogo CMA- Kossodo)

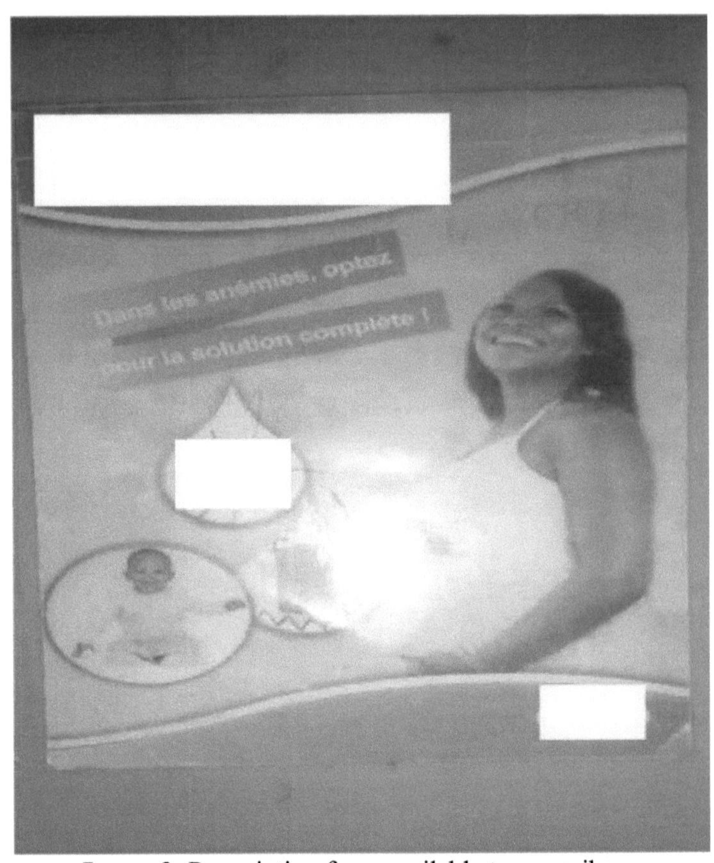

Image 3: Prescription form available to prescribers.
Source (L. Sawadogo CHU-YO)

APPENDICES

Appendix 1: Collection form

I. Socio-professional characteristics of the prescriber

Q1. Age :

Q2. Gender : male/ / female/ /

Q3. Health establishment : CHU-YO/__/CHU-CDG/__/ CHU-B/__/ CHU-T/_/CMA/__/ If CMA specify CMA :

Q4. Professional qualifications: Specialist/__/ DES/__/ General practitioner/__/

Q5. If specialist, please specify :

Q6. years of professional experience :

II. Frequent visits by medical representatives to health centres

Q1. Have you ever received a visit from medical representatives: yes/ / no/ /

Q2. How many visits do you receive per day (in numbers)? :

Q3. How much time do you spend with delegates during a visit (in minutes)? :

Q4. how many laboratories visit you per week (in number)? :

III.Quality of exchanges between medical representatives and doctors

Q1. What was the medical delegate's basic profession: Doctor /__/ Pharmacist/__/ Nurse /__/ Don't know /__/ Other/__/ If other specify :

Q2. Have you ever received presentations from medical delegates: yes/__/ no/__/

Q3. If yes which one(s): Medical equipment / / money / / samples of medication/ / Fuel/ / Catering/ / Conferences/ / Others : / / If other Specify :

Q4. Do you check the information given by the medical representative: Yes/__/ No/__/

Q5. If yes, or would you check the information :
colleagues/__/readings
of articles/ / Other : / / If other, please specify :

Q6 What type of information is collected during the medical check-up?
Dosage/__/ Side effects/__/ Duration of treatment/__/
Shapes/__/ effectiveness /__/price /__/
If form specify Injectables/__/ Tablets /__/ Topicals /__/ Other: /__/

Q7. In your opinion, which class of drugs was most prevalent?

Antibiotic/ / Anti-inflammatory/ / Analgesics/ / Others to be specified: ...

IV. Prescription-related factors

Q1. Approximately how many prescriptions do you write each day?

Do you prescribe DCI/__/ Speciality/__/

Q2. Do you agree that medical representatives influence medical prescribing: Yes/__/No/__/

Q3. Do you agree with the idea that doctors should be accountable to the medical delegates after their visit: Yes/__/No/__/

Q4. Is the visit from the medical representatives your source of information about new medicines? Yes/__/No/__/

Q5. Do you ever prescribe a medicine following a promise of a medical visitor received after a visit from a medical delegate? Yes/ No/ /
Q6 Do you sometimes refuse offers from medical sales representatives: Yes/__/ No/__/
If yes, why?
Q7. What liability may be incurred in the event of the medical representative influencing the medical prescription: Civil /__/ criminal/__/ administrative /__/ disciplinary/__/
Q8. What faults can be attributed to civil liability?
Incorrect prescription/__/incorrect dosage/route of administration/__/ contraindications/__/ failure to monitor/__/
Q9: What types of misconduct can be held criminally liable?
Deliberate failure to observe a duty of safety or **care/__/** infringement of the law on medicinal products/__/ overdosing /__/
Q10 What types of misconduct can be attributed to disciplinary liability?
Non-effective prescription/__/non-qualified prescription/__/non-qualified prescription
security/__/
Q11 When disciplinary liability is incurred, what sanctions are provided for by the Ordre des Médecins?
The warning/__/
Le blame/ /
Temporary deregistration/__/Final deregistration/__/
Appendix 2: Collection authorisation

Appendix 2: Collection authorisation

MINISTERE DE LA SANTE
ET DE L'HYGIENE PUBLIQUE

BURKINA FASO
Unité – Progrès – Justice

REGION DU CENTRE

DIRECTION REGIONALE DE LA SANTE
ET DE L'HYGIENE PUBLIQUE

N°2024/__________/ MS/RCEN/DRSHPC

Ouagadougou, le 08 JAN 2024

AUTORISATION DE COLLECTE

Je soussigné, Directeur régional de la santé et de l'hygiène publique du Centre, autorise Monsieur SAWADOGO Laurent Wendlamita étudiant en thèse de doctorat de Médicine à réaliser dans le cadre de sa thèse une collecte de données sur le thème **«Responsabilités médicales face à l'influence des délégués medicaux dans la prescription médicale en milieu hospitalier»**. La collecte de données de cette étude se déroulera durant le mois de Janvier 2024 et concernera les médecins des districts sanitaires de Baskuy, Bogocogo, Boulmiougou, Nongr-Massom, Sig-Noghin.

Par ailleurs, je vous invite à déposer un exemplaire du rapport de collecte de données à la Direction régionale de la santé et de l'hygiène publique du Centre.

Aussi, le document final validé dans le cadre de cette étude nous sera indispensable pour le service de documentation de notre structure.

La présente autorisation est délivrée sur demande de l'intéressée.

Ampliations

- Districts sanitaires Baskuy, Bogodogo, Boulmiougou, Nongr-Massom, Sig-Noghin
- Archives/chrono

Directeur Régional

Le Directeur Régional

Dr Daniel YERBANGA
Médecin de Santé Publique

MINISTERE DE LA SANTE ET DE L'HYGIENE PUBLIQUE

****

SECRETARIAT GENERAL

BURKINA FASO

******

Unité - Progrès - Justice

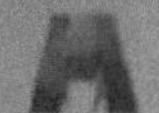

Centre Hospitalier Universitaire Pédiatrique
Charles de Gaulle (CHUP-CDG)
[illegible]

DIRECTION GENERALE

****

DIRECTION DES RESSOURCES HUMAINES

****

N°2024-162/MSHP/SG/CHUP-CDG/DG/DRH/SRF

Ouagadougou, le 17 JAN 2024

La Directrice Générale

A

Monsieur le Docteur W Norbert RAMDE, MCA
Directeur de mémoire.

Objet : autorisation de collecte de données

J'accuse réception de votre lettre dans laquelle vous sollicitez une autorisation de collecte données au profit de **monsieur SAWADOGO Laurent**, étudiante en médecine, dans le cadre de la rédaction d'une thèse dont le thème est « ***Responsabilités médicales face à l'influence des délégués médicaux dans la prescription médicale en milieu hospitalier*** ».

Par la présente, je vous informe que je marque mon accord pour la réalisation de ladite collecte de données dans **le strict respect de l'éthique et de la déontologie dans notre structure**.

Pour les modalités pratiques, je vous invite à prendre attache avec **Monsieur le Professeur Isso OUEDRAOGO, Directeur des services médicaux et techniques (DSMT)**.

Je vous informe dès à présent qu'au terme de son travail, il a l'obligation de déposer **deux (02) exemplaires** du document au **secrétariat particulier** de la Direction générale pour la Bibliothèque du CHUP-CDG.

Tout en vous souhaitant bonne réception, ***recevez Monsieur le Docteur***, mes meilleures salutations.

Cyrille Priscille KABORE/OUEDRAOGO
Chevalier de l'Ordre National
Médaille d'Honneur des Collectivités locales

Ampliations :
1-DRH
1-DSMT
1-DPHUC
1-SRF
1-Intéressé
1-Chronos

MINISTERE DE LA SANTE ET DE L'HYGIENNE PUBLIQUE

SECRETARIAT GENERAL

CENTRE HOSPITALIER UNIVERSITAIRE DE BOGODOGO

DIRECTION GENERALE

N°2024/____/MSHP/SG/CHU-B/DG

BURKINA FASO

Unité-Progrès-Justice

Ouagadougou, le 24 JAN 2024

Le Directeur général

A

Monsieur SAWADOGO Laurant

OUAGADOUGOU

Objet : Autorisation de collecte de données

J'accuse réception de votre lettre à la date du 29 décembre 2023 relative à une autorisation de collecte de données.

Je marque mon accord pour cette demande de collecte de données pour l'étude dont le thème est « **RESPONSABILITES MEDICALES FACE A L'INFLUENCE DES DELEGUES MEDICAUX DANS LA PRESCRIPTION MEDICARE EN MILIEU HOSPITALIER**».

Je vous demande de prendre attache avec le chef de service de la santé publique du Centre Hospitalier Universitaire de Bogodogo pour les aspects pratiques de l'enquête.

Aussi, voudrais-je vous inviter à nous fournir les résultats à la fin de l'étude.

Recevez mes meilleures salutations.

Seydou NOMBRE

Chevalier de l'ordre national

MINISTERE DE LA SANTE ET DE L'HYGIENE PUBLIQUE

SECRETARIAT GENERAL

CENTRE HOSPITALIER UNIVERSITAIRE YALGADO OUEDRAOGO

DIRECTION GENERALE

2023-……MSHP/SG/CHU-YO/DG/DSP

BURKINA FASO

Unité-Progrès-Justice

Ouagadougou, le

LE DIRECTEUR GENERAL

Au

Pr W. Norbert RAMDE

Objet : Autorisation de collecte de données

J'accuse réception de votre demande relative à l'objet ci-dessus par laquelle vous demandez une autorisation de collecte de donnés au profit l'étudiant **SAWADOGO Laurent Wendlamita** dans le cadre de l'élaboration de sa thèse dont le thème «Responsabilités médicales face à l'influence des délégués médicaux dans la prescription médicale en milieu hospitalier»

En réponse, j'ai le plaisir de vous informer que je marque mon accord pour le déroulement de ladite collecte au **CHU-YO.**

Cependant l'étudiant SAWADOGO Laurent Wendlamita est tenu de bien vouloir déposer une copie finale de sa thèse au département de santé publique du CHU-YO.

Pour les modalités pratiques, il voudra bien prendre attache avec les responsables des services concernés.

Tout en vous souhaitant une bonne réception, veuillez recevoir, mes salutations.

Ampliation :

- Intéressé(e)
- DSP
- Tout service

Le Directeur Général par intérim

Pr Georges OUEDRAOGO

Chevalier de l'ordre National

MINISTERE DE L'ENSEIGNEMENT SUPERIEUR, DE LA RECHERCHE, ET DE L'INNOVATION
****
UNIVERSITE JOSEPH KI-ZERBO
****
UNITE DE FORMATION ET DE RECHERCHE EN SCIENCES DE LA SANTE (UFR/SDS)
****
SECTION MEDECINE
****
03 BP : 7021 OUAGADOUGOU 03
TEL : 25-33-73-97 FAX : 25-3373-98

BURKINA FASO
****
Unité - Progrès - Justice

Ouagadougou le 10 mai 2024

ATTESTATION DE CORRECTION

Je soussigné le Docteur Wélébnoaga Norbert RAMDE (MCA), Directeur de Thèse et le Professeur Tarcicius KONSEM, Président du Jury, certifions que le Docteur SAWADOGO Laurent Wendlamita a apporté ses corrections à la thèse intitulée : « responsabilité médicale face à l'influence des délégués médicaux dans la prescription médicale en milieu hospitalier », conformément aux recommandations des membres du Jury.

Le Directeur de Thèse

Ramdé

Dr Wélébnoaga Norbert RAMDE (MCA)

Le Président du Jury

Docteur KONSEM Tarcissus
Stomatologiste et Chirurgien
Maxillo- Facial
Professeur Titulaire

Pr Tarcicius KONSEM

HIPPOCRATIC OATH

In the presence of the teachers of this school and my dear fellow students, I promise and swear to be faithful to the laws of honour and probity in the practice of medicine. I will give my free care to the needy and I will never demand a salary above my work. Admitted to the interior of houses, my eyes will not see what goes on there; my tongue will keep silent about the secrets entrusted to me and my status will not be used to corrupt morals or encourage crime. Respectful and grateful to my masters, I will give back to their children the education I received from their fathers. May men esteem me if I remain faithful to my promises. May I be shamed and despised by my colleagues if I fail to do so.

SUMMARY

Title: Medical responsibility and the influence of medical representatives on medical prescribing in hospitals.

Objective: To study medical responsibility in relation to the influence of medical representatives on medical prescribing in hospitals.

Method: This was a descriptive cross-sectional study with prospective collection carried out in the public hospitals of Ouagadougou from 08 January to 31 January 2024. A self-administered form was proposed to the doctors.

Results: Our study involved 213 doctors in the city of Ouagadougou, with an average prescriber age of 34.7 years and a male predominance of 58.7%. Doctors specialising in this field were the most represented (51.2%). The proportion of doctors with less than 5 years' professional experience was 50%. 95.8% of prescribers said they had received gifts, most of which were samples of medicines 91.8% of medical equipment 87.1% catering 39.7% conference funding 39.2% .... The Internet was the most common source of information used (44.1%) by prescribers to check the information provided by the medical representative. Antibiotics were the most common class of medication (62.3%), with 66% of prescribers being specialists. Doctors (81.7%) acknowledged the influence on their prescribing. Knowledge of doctors' responsibilities showed that the majority of prescribers (78.88%) had a good knowledge of their prescribing responsibilities.

Conclusion : Doctors are influenced by the medical visit and have average knowledge of prescribing responsibility.

Key words: Responsibility for prescribing; influence; medical representative; prescriber.

Author : SAWADOGO Laurent Wendlamita **Email** : laurentsa3 @gmail .com

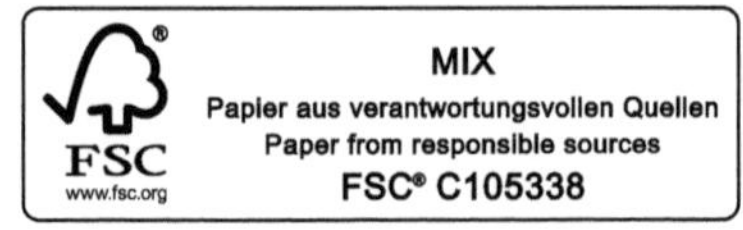

Printed by Books on Demand GmbH, Norderstedt / Germany